Leaky Gut

The Beginners Guide to Healing Your Digestive Tract

Thank you for spending your hard-earned money on purchasing a copy of this book. We sincerely wish it helps you make positive steps in your health journey!

Table of Contents

Introduction

In this book, you will learn about a growing, yet often overlooked, medical concern many people experience today. Leaky gut syndrome is something that can affect anyone and many people struggle with, whether they know about it or not.

Chronic stress, poor diet, medications, and toxins are just some of the causes and also something that is prevalent in today's society. No matter where you go, we are confronted with tempting processed foods.

A ride home after a tough day of work features a slew of restaurants filled with greasy, salty and sugary foods. A stroll down most grocery store aisles proves that most are stuffed with boxed, bagged and canned foods pumped with sugar, preservatives, chemicals, colorings, and flavorings while being processed into a health-destroying time bomb. Even some of the food that we would normally deem healthy is covered in pesticides, filled with hormones and antibiotics, or is genetically modified. If the food repels and kills bugs, imagine what it does to our digestion systems. If the animal required antibiotics, is it really something we should be eating anyway?

Food is our fuel and we need to pay attention to what we're putting into the machine that is our body. Not to mention, on top of the damaging foods we're offered, we work long and often arduous hours, surrounded by stressful situations, staggering debts, and constantly dinging cell phones. It's no wonder our guts and ultimately our immune systems are exhausted, weak, and deprived.

The following chapters will discuss how to take your diagnosis, or even suspicion of leaky gut and conquer it! No longer will you feel helpless after a meal, dealing with the symptoms of a damaged GI tract.

Learn about what can make your condition worse, what will help it and get a comprehensive plan to cure your digestion. Through simple and basic foods, you will immediately see progress. Many of the cures featured in this book are ones you can make or find easily and cheaply. No more taking mystery pills hoping that they don't end up causing more issues down the road. The old saying, 'You are what you eat,' could not be any truer!

Also, learn about some herbal remedies to incorporate into your diet to help heal and soothe damaged tissues and linings. Then check out some extra supplements to try to really kick the healing into hyperdrive!

Overall, leaky gut is a condition that can be stopped. You can take charge of your own health without relying on medicines from a pharmacy. Instead get your cure from a FARMacy! Start eating basic, organic, pesticide-free foods and see the results right away. No more migraines, fatigue, joint pain, bloat, digestion problems, stomach pain, or skin issues. Plus, no more weight gain and with some exercise, you will be feeling better than ever, your confidence will shoot up, you will feel happier and be able to handle stress better. Stop chasing down dead ends and do something today that can make a huge difference in your life!

There are plenty of books on this subject on the market, thanks again for choosing this one! Every effort was made to ensure it is full of as much useful information as possible, please enjoy!

Chapter 1:
What Exactly is Leaky Gut?

It's hard these days to maintain a healthy diet, what with GMOs, preservatives, and processed foods flooding the aisles in almost every grocery store. Add that with the lack of information up until a few short years ago, and it's no wonder people are developing health issues. One of these issues is called leaky gut syndrome, and it's still somewhat of a mystery in the medical field.

Our digestive tract is one of the biggest parts of our immune system and can tip the scales from healthy to unhealthy. Being told you have leaky gut isn't really the end result of some specific cause, rather it's more of the beginning to a rocky road. Having a leaky gut can lead to much more serious health diseases if not treated. In itself, a leaky gut will have symptoms of cramps, bloating, food sensitivities, gas, and aches and pain. First, let's talk about what exactly a leaky gut is.

Intestinal Permeability

Leaky gut is also known as intestinal permeability, Hyper-permeable intestines, or dysbiosis. It is a condition where the lining of the small intestine is damaged and is porous, thus causing undigested food, bacteria and toxic waste to flow, or leak, through the intestines and spill into the blood stream.

When it gets into the blood stream, the body interprets them as foreign particles and enacts an autoimmune response which includes, inflammation and allergic reactions like migraines, IBS or Irritable Bowel Syndrome, rheumatoid arthritis, eczema, food allergies, chronic fatigue, and more. The damaged cells in the intestines do not generate the enzymes needed to properly digest the food. As a result, your body won't get to absorb the nutrients which leads to a weakened immune system and hormone imbalances.

Our intestines are our first guard in our immune system. The outermost layer of intestinal cells, or epithelial, connect to frames called tight junctions. At the ends of the junctions are the microvilli. They absorb correctly digested nutrients and move them through the epithelial cells to the bloodstream. With a healthy digestion procedure, the tight junctions are closed, which forces the molecules flowing by to be screened, allowing only the properly digested particles to pass through via the mucosa cells, much like the TSA at the airport.

With a damaged intestine, undigested particles slip through and enter the blood stream. The body recognizes something isn't right and see the particles as foreign bodies. First, the liver kicks into gear and works overtime to filter the blood removing the particles as best as it can. In most situations, the liver can't keep up with the constant flow of waste, so they start accumulating in the body. Then the immune system gets called to action and attacks the particles. Still, particles get away and they rest in the body's tissue.

This causes inflammation which in turn creates more stress for the immune system. At this point, the body is fighting a war and smaller more insignificant jobs are getting ignored like calming the inflammation, fighting bacteria, regulating the gut and so on. This can lead to MS, ulcerative colitis, IBS, chronic fatigue, and fibromyalgia.

The body will start to create antibody soldiers to fight the same foreign particles that they originally fought in the first attack whenever they enter the body, which can range from phenols, proteins, casein protein, and glycerin. After a long period of time with a leaky gut, the body will prepare with the antibodies whenever it detects them again. If you have food sensitivities to more than a dozen foods, you might have a leaky gut.

Any of the undigested food that leaks into the gut is now considered an enemy and will create a reaction from your immune system.

Core Causes of Leaky Gut

Below are some of the main causes of a leaky gut. While the causes are still debated in the medical community, there are some basic contributors to the damage created in the intestine.

Bad Diet

Eating too many processed foods, refined sugars, refined flours, preservatives, chemicals, colorings, and flavorings can create a leaky gut. All these chemicals are toxic to the body and can build up making the body have to work harder and harder until it can't keep up.

Chronic Stress

Stress will repress the immune system. Your body can't differentiate between a life-threatening situation and getting a shut-off notice from the electric company, so it enacts the same flight or fight response no matter what. This stops lesser functions from happening, focuses on those needed to either fight or escape, and floods the body with energizing hormones. In a life-threatening situation, this response is a life saver, in an emotional on non-life threatening situation, the hormones go unused and wreak havoc on the body. If this happens a lot, the body is constantly interrupted and won't function properly. It weakens the immune system and is overrun very quickly.

Bad Bacteria and Toxins

We all have healthy and beneficial bacteria in our guts. It's what makes our systems stronger, helps along our digestion and counterbalances bad bacteria and pathogens. If the bad outweighs the good, the pathogens take over and inflame the membranes in the intestines, eventually making it porous. The same goes for toxins, if there is too much present in the digestion, or is chronically present, it can overwhelm the digestion process and wear on the protective lining.

Other Possible Causes

Inflammation in the gut from other factors can cause leaky gut. Other factors might be low stomach acid, bacteria overgrowth, yeast overgrowth, parasites, infection, and excessive environmental toxins.

Certain medications, whether they are over the counter or prescribed, can irritate the stomach lining and decrease the mucosal levels (the gastrointestinal tract's protective lining).

Excessive yeast build up can mutate into multi-called fungus such as candida. It will grow many arms that reach out and cling to the intestinal lining eventually making holes in it. Yeast is a normal occurrence in the stomach, but too much is a problem.

Zinc helps maintain the strength of the mucosal lining, and a deficiency in zinc will leave the body with a weak lining, eventually leading to its deterioration and permeation.

Many of the symptoms of a leaky gut are shared with other illnesses. They are not unique and can be misinterpreted. Therefore, it is important to find a doctor that appreciates your concerns and will take the time to see a diagnosis through to the end in case it was wrong or didn't fully take care of the issue.

Common Symptoms

Some common symptoms are:

- Food allergies or sensitivities
- Bloating
- Thyroid conditions
- IBS (Irritable Bowel Syndrome)
- Joint pain
- Chronic fatigue
- Headaches and migraines
- Digestive problems such as diarrhea, constipation, and excessive gas
- Autism
- Mood issues or imbalances
- Weight gain
- Skin issues like rosacea, psoriasis, eczema, and acne
- Nutritional deficiencies
- Poor immune system
- Brain fog and memory loss
- Carbohydrate and sugar cravings
- Arthritis and joint pain
- Depression, ADD, ADHD, and anxiety
- Autoimmune conditions such as rheumatoid arthritis, celiac disease, lupus, and Crohn's disease

Again, many of these symptoms are caused by different illnesses as well, so it's important to pay attention to your symptoms as well as when and how they occur. Keep a diary of them, when they happen, what you ate prior to the occurrence and so on. Bring your notes with you to your next doctor's appointment.

When it's all boiled down, leaky gut syndrome is a broad condition with many possible causes and many possible symptoms. It seems to be mainly affected by what we eat and recently may be the root cause of a lot of different illnesses. With our modern diets and daily mental stressors, leaky gut appears to be a common condition that is often overlooked.

Chapter 2:
Home Remedies

Now that you know what leaky gut is, some of its symptoms and a few of its major causes, how can it be cured?

Most of the causes of a leaky gut are food related, so a cure must also be in the food. As mentioned earlier, the food that is available today is often filled with preservatives, coloring or flavoring, sugars, and chemicals. Processed foods fill the shelves and what would be considered healthy food is often covered in pesticides, filled with antibiotics and hormones or is genetically modified from its natural state. These are not the type of foods that anyone should be using as fuel.

Also try to eat foods that are wild caught, organically grown, and are raised without hormones or antibiotics. Eat meat from healthy and humanely raised animals or wild caught or hunted animals. Eat fruits, vegetables, and grains that were not sprayed with pesticides or genetically modified. Locally grown and raised foods are the best and are usually the most reliable. However, in the recent years, the public has been more conscious about where their food comes from and therefore whole foods stores, organic sections and farmers markets have become more and more common and easily accessible.

Besides doing this, here are some foods to incorporate into your diet to help soothe and heal a leaky gut.

Water

Water is life and is crucial to every single process in the body. The digestion tract is no different and relies on water to break down, digest and utilize nutrients from the food. If you don't drink enough water throughout the day, you become dehydrated. Chronic dehydration will allow the waste matter in your gut to harden and become stagnate.

Next, bad bacteria will take over and inflame the lining of the stomach, creating a leaky gut. To avoid this, drink plenty of water. Some doctors say to drink at least 8 glasses of water a day while others say to only drink when you are thirsty.

Regardless of which you chose, try to only drink water throughout the day. Other beverages can dehydrate you rather than help you, some are filled with sugars which should be avoided anyways, and others can irritate your bowels putting stress on the GI tract and immune system. If you already have bowel issues, drink a couple extra glasses of water to help your body digest your food better.

One way to kick your water consumption up a notch is to add organic apple cider vinegar. Apple cider vinegar is a fermented tonic that is anti-microbial and kills bad bacteria such as H Pylori. This type of bacteria can cause stomach ulcers and acid reflux. The tonic is also packed full of organic acids and enzymes that actually improve the digestion process, reduce inflammation in the body and stabilize blood sugar levels. Mix 1-2 tablespoons of apple cider vinegar into at least 8 ounces of water or drizzle onto meat and vegetable dishes. Also, the acids in apple cider vinegar help pre-digest the foods, which help reduce the stress load on your own digestion. It improves the creation and flow of digestive juices such as bile, stomach acid, and pancreatic enzymes as well. Try to use 3-4 tablespoons of apple cider vinegar a day, whether it is in water or on your meat and vegetables.

Ginger

Ginger is a very effective treatment for leaky gut and it can easily be incorporated into daily meals. It compliments Asian cuisine and many baked goods. It does well in casseroles and on chicken as well. You can also chew on a small chunk of ginger or make it into a tea.

Ginger reduces inflammation and irritation in the lining of the intestines. It also has powerful anti-oxidant components that rid the gastrointestinal tract of bad bacteria, toxins, and other microorganisms. This reduces the amount that is leaked into the blood stream.

Garlic

Garlic reduces blood pressure and cholesterol levels in the body. It also removes excessive yeast from the stomach and intestines. Eating a few cloves of raw garlic a day efficiently treats a leaky gut. Adding garlic to everyday meals helps heal the intestines and balance out the bacteria in the stomach, reducing the reoccurrence of bad bacteria leaking into the blood. It also lowers the risk of heart disease and can subdue the growth of a tumor.

Garlic brings almost every type of meat to life and fills it with great flavor. It can be used for most styles and types of cuisines and can be sprinkled or added to all types of vegetable dishes, soups, casseroles, breakfasts, and sandwiches or salads.

Bone Broth

Bone broth is exactly as it sounds, it is a broth or soup made by boiling bones from chicken or other fowl, beef and other red meat animals, fish with water. This seemingly simple food item is very beneficial to both the leaky gut syndrome as well as the rest of the body. It also helps diseases such as arthritis and autoimmunity since it contains nutrients that help heal any damaged skin, heal joints, support the immune system, decrease inflammation, and heal intestinal cells.

Some of the nutrients present in bone broth are amino acids in the protein, which is released during the cooking process. Glutamine is one that is mainly used by the small intestinal cells. When you get stressed out, glutamine is used up and your cells in your small intestine become deficient. When you replace the glutamine taken, the intestinal cells get what they need to be healthy and eventually start repairing themselves. Arginine and proline are anti-inflammatory. Glycine calms the nervous system while supporting a balanced stomach acid and helps bile secretion needed to digest the food in the GI tract. This nutrient is also significant to the liver and is needed to make an anti-oxidant called glutathione. Glycine is also known to be an anti-inflammatory. Cysteine helps to thin out any mucus. It can also be used to make the anti-oxidant called glutathione. All of this put together makes for a leaky gut remedy that decreases oxidative stress and autoimmunity.

Bone broth also offers a matrix called collagen that gets broken down transforming into gelatin. It is the same stuff used to make jello products, and if you were to make bone broth and then put it in the fridge, the next day you will find giggling, bouncing bone jello! Gelatin helps heal the lining in the intestines because it supports mucus production and in turn, protects the intestinal cells. Without the protective layer of mucus in the intestines, the cells would be exposed to bad bacteria that would eat up the lining and create holes in it. Gelatin is another nutrient that is anti-inflammatory which helps the body heal. When it is absorbed into the body, gelatin can be used in several areas in the body such as the skin, your nails, and your hair.

Glycosaminoglycans contain glucosamine, hyaluronic acid, and chondroitin that help heal arthritis and joint pain. When you boil down the bones, the cartilage present in the joints breaks down and releases the glycosaminoglycans into the broth. You could take a pill form supplement to get all of these, or you can add bone broth into your normal cooking recipes and reap the benefits of all the nutrients it has to offer.

Bone broth also has some minerals to offer. These minerals include magnesium, calcium, phosphorus, potassium, silica, and other trace minerals (for instance fish bones have iodine in them). These are all as helpful as electrolytes which keep you hydrated and support bone health. The electrolytes are important for cell function, including intestinal cells. The marrow in the bones has been used for centuries and has been thought to also support a healthy immune system.

To make bone broth, you will need about 12 to 72 hours, a large pot, fresh bones, and water. Get bones from your choice of meat, whether that is beef, chicken, fowl, fish and so on. Try to use bones that are from healthy animals that have been grass fed and raised either wild or humanely, preferably with no hormones or antibiotics used either. The bones don't need to be perfect either. They can have some meat or seasonings on them. You can use feet or hooves, heads or skulls, necks, tails and many other seemingly inedible parts of the animal. Just be sure that the parts you use are clean. You don't want to incorporate old bedding, dirt, or feces into your soup.

Place the bones into a large pot then fill it with water until the bones are covered. Add a couple tablespoons full of apple cider vinegar, this will help pull the nutrients out of the bones. You can also add the inedible parts of vegetables like carrot tops, onion peels, stems, celery butts, garlic peels, carrot peels, as well as any herbs you want such as parsley, basil, rosemary, pepper, thyme, cumin, paprika, and so on. Bring to a boil and lower heat to a simmer for at least 1 to 2 hours if you have sensitive digestion, up to 12 hours with fish bones, and all the way up to 72 hours to really get the most out of the bones.

Add water as needed so it doesn't burn up and cover with a lid with a little gap in the seal. Once you are done boiling and the bones are soft, strain out all the bones and other ingredients. Compost the solids and pour broth into a clean pot. Some people prefer to refrigerate the broth and skim the fat off the top. This really isn't necessary as the fats are beneficial. You can use the broth as is in soups, stews, casseroles, and many other dishes. You can also boil the broth down until is in a concentrated form (about ¼ of the amount of liquid) then disperse it into ice cube trays. After freezing the cubes, pour them into bags and label them with the type of bone broth you made. When you cook, drop a cube right into the pan or mix with a cup of hot water to make 1 cup of broth.

One downfall of bone broth is that it isn't suitable for vegetarians. However, you can make a broth out of beets, seaweed, kale, and spinach to get collagen.

Another concern when making bone broth is that when pulling out the nutrients, toxins from the animals' environment may also leach into the broth. This is why it is best to use bones from healthy animals that were raised without antibiotics and hormones as well as grass fed, or wild caught animals.

Raw Cultured Dairy

If you can tolerate dairy, raw dairy can be very beneficial. When it comes to people who experience a milk sensitivity, they are usually intolerant towards the casein, and more commonly the A1 beta-casein. There are two types of casein, A1 beta-casein, and A2 beta-casein. A1 beta-casein is from newer breeds of cows as opposed to the heritage cows, goats or sheep. If you are or know someone that is intolerant of the A1 beta-casein, they should be okay with goat's milk, sheep's milk, and heritage breeds of cows like Guernsey cows or Jersey cows. Some people, however, are lactose intolerant and need to be careful with all dairy.

If you are the type that can normally handle dairy, yogurt is a healing food. Try to make your own yogurt or find yogurt that still has the culture in it. Most mainstream yogurts are filled with sugar and are pasteurized which takes all the beneficial bacteria and cultures out of them. There is nothing really helpful left in these types of yogurts for a leaky gut. The type you want to find will have a label on it that states there is live cultures in the yogurt.

Colostrum is another type of super dairy product worth trying. It is packed full with secretory IgA (the main immunoglobulin in mucus secretions) and other immunoglobulins that restore an immunity deficient gut. It is better if combined with a probiotic. Colostrum has a small amount of lactose, so if you are lactose intolerant or sensitive, try a small amount first or try it with a probiotic to see if you can manage it. It is usually tolerated well by most people with this condition. If you are casein sensitive, try a goat colostrum first, especially if you don't know which type of casein you are sensitive to. You can find it in powder form at many stores, but you can also go to a farm and ask for the colostrum from the first three milkings of the cow, goat, or sheep.

As for fermented dairy, most regions in the world have their own version of it. The people of Bulgaria have yogurt, the people of India have lassi, the people of Africa have amasi, and the people of Eastern Russia and Slovakia have kefir. All of these products were mixed with a lactic acid originating from bacteria like Lactococcus, Leuconostoc, or Lactobacillus to ferment the food. These raw, fermented foods have many of the same bacterial strains in them such as the lactic acid based lactobacillus family of kefir, bulgaricus, parakefir, casei, brevis, and so on. These are all good bacteria that will balance out the gut.

These products also provide the healthy type of yeast, saccharomyces, for the gut such as saccharomyces unisporus, cerevisiae, turicensis, and exiguous varieties. Finally, raw fermented dairy products contain one of the best and most vigorous strains of probiotics, bacillus coagulans. All of these cultures combine to work together to protect and repair the gut. They also destroy the bad bacteria and even the most opportunistic organism like the Candida yeast variety. Altogether a powerful punch to the bad organisms in the gut.

Fermented Vegetables

Same as the fermented dairy, fermented vegetables are amazing for the gastrointestinal tract. Any fermented or cultured food is important to the gut not only for the probiotic contents but also for the micro- and macronutrients that are enriched and the fact that they are easily digested and absorbed into the body.

When most people hear cultured food they think of yogurt, but there are many other cultured foods as well. Cultured vegetables can be kimchi or sauerkraut, cultured fruits include preserved fruits and chutneys, cultured beverages include beet kvass, kombucha, and water kefir, cultured grains are foods like sourdough bread and cakes, cultured dairy products include kefir, creme fraiche, yogurt, and sour cream, and cultured condiments include fish sauce, ketchup, fermented salsa, soy sauce or tamari, and so on.

These are all foods that can be naturally fermented and turned into a super version of itself that is both beneficial and tasty! They provide the body with live bioactive enzymes, good microorganisms, B vitamins, and organic acids. These nutrients enhance the digestive functions in the body by invigorating the creation of the proper amount of stomach acid levels, pancreatic enzymes and bile secretions for an ideal digestion.

To start healing a leaky gut, try to consume around 4 ounces of fermented drinks and 4 ounces of fermented vegetables a day. Start slowly at first, only consume about 2 or 3 tablespoons at a time and increase every other day by a tablespoon at a time. Eventually, you will get to 4 ounces a day each and if you enjoy the drinks of foods, you can eat or drink more. If you develop any rashes or indigestion from the food, slow down or take a break for a couple days. Too much, too fast may cause bloating or diarrhea.

Some tasty examples to try are:

- Beet kvass
- Kimchi
- Yogurt
- Kefir
- Coconut milk kefir / Coconut water kefir
- Sauerkraut
- Fermented vegetables or soy
- Kombucha
- Apple cider vinegar

Coconut

Coconut products have grown in popularity lately and for good reason. Coconuts are one of the most multi-functional and healthiest foods on our planet. They are popular for the following reasons:

- Antibacterial & antimicrobial properties
- Enhances digestion, intestinal health, and nutrient absorption into the body
- Health benefits for the cardiovascular system
- Contains anti-cancer properties
- Treats and manages diabetes
- Helps against HIV/AIDS
- Helps, manages, or rids the brain of various neurological disorders
- Supports your immune system
- Improves liver and kidney health
- Enhances athletic performance

- Helps manage your metabolism, energy and weight management

Not only does it help in all these regions, coconut products are also sources of medium chain triglycerides. These reduce inflammation, help burn fat, and heal the lining of the gut. Coconut oil is packed with lauric acid which can be found in high quantities in breast milk. It's known as a potent anti-microbial agent that conquers bad yeast and bad bacteria.

Used as a natural and healthy skin moisturizer, it can also be eaten in a wide variety of meals. When applied topically it still enters the blood stream where it can positively affect multiple body functions. Try to use about 3 or 4 tablespoons a day. Coconut butter has all the same benefits as coconut oil but the addition of coconut flour, which is where all the fiber is located. The flour supports and feeds a healthy microbiome and is a great prebiotic. Coconut butter is amazing in desert type of meals and savory type of dishes.

Sprouted Seeds

Some people may have problems eating and digesting beans, nuts, grains and seeds, they may even cause more inflammation. Sprouting these kernels adds helpful and healing enzymes as well as making it easier for the digestion system to break down and absorb it. It also enhances the helpful gut flora amounts in the GI tract, which in turn decreases the autoimmune reactions to the grains, nut, seeds, and beans of all types. Especially when it comes to grains. Many people struggle to digest grains, but by sprouting them and then eating the sprouts, it breaks down the complex starches and sugars before, making them easier to absorb. Now it's pretty easy to come across sprouted seeds to purchase You could find everything from chia seeds to flax seeds, to possibly even hemp. Not to mention the plethora of other nuts and grains available.

Some research shows that grain sprouts are easier to break down and digest for people who suffer from diabetes because the sprouts have a different and more manageable amount of phenolic acids and enzymes accessible. Both the long and short term sprouting allowed diabetics to level out their amylase-enzyme levels, which is necessary to normally digest glucose. More research will be beneficial but it may be a way for people with insulin resistance to digest and utilize the sugars in any high glycemic foods. More research is needed for fermented grains like sourdough as well.

Leaky gut is often caused by a poor diet and bad choices in today's grocery stores. Like many digestion issues, by first choosing better food options, the body will get a chance to heal itself and get a boost of many beneficial nutrients to help it along.

Chapter 3:
Supplementary Natural Remedies

Once you have started eating healthier and are more aware of the foods you eat and how they affect you, you can start to initiate other means to healing your body.

Eating the right foods keeps toxins, chemicals, GMOs, and processed foods from damaging your system further, and there are some herbs and supplements that can help you heal your body faster.

Below is a list of herbs and supplements to try out. Remember to start slow and take a minimum amount until you know your body can handle the new remedy and then slowly increase the amount.

Peppermint Tea

Peppermint is a wonderful herb that is beneficial for many stomach and digestion issues such as leaky gut. It promotes bile secretion to improve digestion and when taken in tea form, it soothes the intestinal walls while wiping out the bad bacteria and toxins in the intestines. This prevents many of them from leaking and lowers the infection, thereby lessening the symptoms associated with a leaky gut. Two glasses a day of this tea can help heal a leaky gut. A peppermint oil capsule is believed to have the same benefits as well.

Chamomile Tea

Chamomile tea is known to help a leaky gut. Chamomile reduces symptoms such as bloating, cramps, flatulence, and stomach pain as it is a natural relaxant. The herb also naturally reduces mental stress and anxiety which in turn negates the stress response system in the body that lowers the immune system needed to deal with leaked particles.

Slippery Elm

Slippery elm is normally used to treat wounds, burns, and various other skin inflammations, but if taken orally it helps soothe inflamed intestines. When slippery elm is mixed with water it becomes a gelatinous court of substance that easily coats the lining of the intestines, soothing and strengthening it. Plus, the antioxidants in slippery elm fight off free radicals.

L-Glutamine

L-glutamine is an amino acid that consists up to 35 percent of the body's amino acid nitrogen in the blood. It is a building block for protein and is widely used throughout the body. The body uses it a lot so it is considered an essential amino acid. L-glutamine enhances the gastrointestinal tract as it is an important nutrient for the intestines to repair itself and it protects against further damage. It also can heal ulcers. It can improve diarrhea and IBS by balancing out the mucus creation and enhances cellular detoxification and metabolism.

Not only is it good for the gut, it also is an essential neurotransmitter for the brain that helps with focus, memory, and concentration. It can promote muscle growth and endurance while curbing any cravings for sugar and alcohol. On top of all that, L-glutamine fights cancer and improves blood sugar and diabetes. Overall a great supplement to help treat leaky gut as well as general health.

Quercetin

Quercetin acts like an antihistamine with its anti-inflammatory properties. It also improves the GI tract's barrier functions by helping to seal the lining. It does this by producing tight junction proteins for the body's use.

Licorice Root

Licorice root increases the availability of hormones while relieving adrenal fatigue since it helps the body absorb and metabolize cortisol. It also upholds the body's creation and maintenance of the mucosal lining of the gut. It can be especially beneficial if a leaky gut was caused by emotional stress. Licorice root has glycyrrhizin in it which can cause hypertension and edema. It would be a good idea to find a de-glycyrrhizinated licorice or DGL.

Digestive Enzymes

Digestive enzymes help break down any proteins, starches, and complex sugars that may be in a meal. This will help reduce intestinal inflammation and make the food easier to digest and utilize. Take them before and after a meal, especially one that may not be filled with the best ingredients. Try to find a supplement that has at least these components in it:

- Protease – digests proteins (as well as gluten)
- Lipase – digests fats
- Amylase – digests starches
- Lactase – digests lactose in dairy

Probiotics

When it comes to probiotics, some improve the immune system while others enhance general health and hormonal balance. Therefore, it's always a good idea to specifically look into each strain before taking them as a supplement. You will maximize your healing and be strategic in doing so.

When you are researching keep track of the genus, species, and strain names. The labels will also tell you the type of colony forming units or CFU's that are around at the time of manufacturing. When you find the right strains, keep in mind the brand quality, the level of CFU's (you want at least 15 billion CFU's), the strain diversity (you want multiple bacterial strains), and the survivability.

Look for strains such as:

- Bifidobacterium bifidum
- Saccharomyces boulardii
- Bifidobacterium longum

- Bacillus coagulans
- Bifidobacterium breve
- Bacillus subtilis
- Lactobacillus bulgaricus
- Bifidobacterium infantis
- Lactobacillus rhamnosus
- Lactobacillus casei
- Lactobacillus brevis
- Lactobacillus acidophilus

Digestion Bitter Tincture

Digestion bitters in the form of tinctures help relieve any indigestion immediately. They also help repair the gut lining and help preserve it. Take ½ - 1 teaspoon before and after each meal or by directions on the label. You can buy them online or in stores like Swedish Bitters or you can make your own at home. Here are some recipes to make your own:

Digestion Bitter #1

4 parts fennel
2 parts dandelion root
2 parts artichoke leaf
2 parts organically cultivated gentian
1 part ginger

Step 1: Combine the herbs and place in a jar
Step 2: Seal jar with lid
Step 3: Shake vigorously once per day
Step 4: Repeat step 3 every day for 6 weeks

Strain into a separate jar after 6 weeks. This mixture will keep indefinitely.

Digestion Bitter #2

20 grams elecampane, dried
10 grams roasted dandelion root, dried
10 grams fresh minced ginger
5 grams licorice root
3 cloves
3 grams cracked black pepper
1 orange
1 vanilla bean pod

Step 1: Put the minced ginger, roots, licorice, pepper and cloves into at least a quart sized jar
Step 2: Cut the whole orange up and put it into the jar
Step 3: Cut open the vanilla bean pod, then mince it finely and add it to the jar as well
Step 4: Pour fresh water into the jar until it covers the herbs
Step 5: Cover it with a lid and then shake it well

Keep it on the counter or a shelf, and shake it occasionally. Two to six weeks later, strain it and put into a clean jar. It will keep indefinitely.

Collagen

Collagen is essential to healing your leaky gut, not only because it's great on its own, which it is, but because it helps boost the effects of proline and glycine, two amino acids. It is mostly used to aid your stomach in producing its mucous lining and gastric juices.

Collagen is often found in broths and can also be purchased as a powdered supplement. This makes for a very simple solution to helping cure leaky gut.

Chapter 4:
Exercise, exercise, exercise!

The other side of this coin to healing your leaky gut is to exercise regularly. Exercise not only uses up the excessive amount of hormones released into the body when the stress response system is activated, it also modifies the inflammation in the body. While exercise can be inflammatory in the short term, in the long run, it is powerfully anti-inflammatory. Researchers have shown that low physical activity leads to more digestion problems.

However, any physical activity in itself should not be stressful. One study with mice found that when the researchers forced the mice to run on a treadmill the mice got worsening symptoms of digestion problems and inflammation increased. The mice that were allowed to run on the treadmill whenever they wanted had a lower amount of inflammation and had no intestinal damage. Thus, if the exercise in itself became a stressor, then it had no effect on healing digestion issues or on inflammation in the gastrointestinal tract.

Another study found that exercise helps reduce gut inflammation and improve gut flora. During a 12-week exercise program, participants had reduced symptoms of indigestion and other stomach issues which suggests the exercise helped the food travel through the digestion tract more efficiently. Exercise also helped manage stress, therefore not inhibiting digestion and the immune system. Exercise can also change the gut flora for the better, setting the balance of good and bad bacteria back to normal. It can also keep up the balance of the microbiome during an episode of stress.

Having a regular exercise program is important, but make sure the act of exercising isn't forced or stressful. One type of exercise that is especially beneficial for a leaky gut is yoga. It is a calming and slow type of exercise that utilizes both body and mind to bring about balance. A lot of gut disorders benefit from this variety of exercise since stress affects the immune system which is mainly located in the gut.

Another type of beneficial exercise is walking. The same study that found yoga to be helpful also found walking to help heal the gut. Walking in itself isn't a stressful type of exercise and it improves the mood, the symptoms from the GI tract, and any anxiety. Plus, both of these types of exercises can be done virtually anywhere.

On the following pages are a few different exercise programs you could follow.

Try to do them around the same time every day and if you find that one type of exercise isn't working out for you, switch it for a different variety.

If none of these work for you try doing something that you think would be fun. Just remember to start out any new exercise slow, gradually increase, and switch it up.

For instance, don't run every single day, or weight train every single day. Your body needs time to heal in between exercising the same muscle groups.

Also, don't start a running program by immediately running 5 miles. Going too far, or too fast right out the gates is a sure-fire way to get an injury, which will lead to more stress.

Exercise Program #1: *Family Program*

Monday:
Leisurely walk around your neighborhood with the family or the dogs (at least 30 minutes)

Tuesday:
Yoga or stretching routine (instructions can easily be found online via Google search, YouTube videos, or at a gym) (30 minutes)

Wednesday:
Leisurely walk around your neighborhood with the family or the dogs (at least 30 minutes)

Thursday:
Bodyweight exercises (pushups, sit-ups, pullups, lunges, stretches etc.) (30 minutes)

Friday:
Fun indoor exercises (dancing, charades, twister, active videogames such as Nintendo Wii, play piggy back rides with the kids etc.) (30-60 minutes)

Saturday:
Outdoor chores like mowing and gardening or raking leaves or shoveling snow or playing outside with the dogs or the kids

Sunday:
Get the family and friends out to play a game of football or baseball, ice skating, sledding, fort building and so on

Exercise Program #2: *Social/Personal Program*

Monday:
Go swimming, alone or with friends, at the local gym

Tuesday:
Walk for 30-60 minutes (depending on your comfortability)

Wednesday:
Solo sports practice (i.e. cycling, skiing, martial arts, boxing, basketball, etc.)

Thursday:
Running/jogging for 30 minutes

Friday:
Yoga or stretching routine (instructions can easily be found online via Google search, YouTube videos, or at a gym)
(30 minutes)

Saturday:
Team sports practice (i.e. tennis, softball, badminton, football, volleyball, basketball, etc.)

Sunday:
Walk for 30-60 minutes (depending on your comfortability)

Exercise Program #3: *Winter Program*

Monday:
Walk for 30-60 minutes outside or inside (depending on your comfortability)

Tuesday:
Sledding, ice skating, snowboarding, cross country ski, snowshoeing or simply playing in the snow for 30 minutes

Wednesday:
Bodyweight exercises (pushups, sit-ups, pullups, lunges, stretches etc.) (30 minutes)

Thursday:
Yoga or stretching routine (instructions can easily be found online via Google search, YouTube videos, or at a gym)
(30 minutes)

Friday:
Fun indoor exercises (dancing, charades, twister, active videogames such as Nintendo Wii, play piggy back rides with the kids etc.) (30-60 minutes)

Saturday: Shovel snow, clean the back/front garden or go for a refreshing walk outside to get your blood pumping

Sunday:
Free choice day, make it at least 30 minutes

Exercise Program #4 *Summer Program*

Monday:
Leisurely walk around the local park for 60 minutes

Tuesday:
Swimming for at least 30 minutes

Wednesday:
Mow the lawn, gardening, raking leaves, washing the car, or any other outdoor chores for 30 minutes

Thursday:
Running/jogging for 30 minutes

Friday:
Team or solo sports practice (i.e. tennis, softball, badminton, football, volleyball, basketball, cycling, etc.)

Saturday:
Swimming or yoga at the beach/gym for 30 minutes

Sunday:
Go hiking or bike riding for at least 60-90 minutes depending on the difficulty

Exercise Program #5: *City/Urban Program*

Monday:
Solo exercise at home (Yoga, Zumba, Thai Chi, CrossFit, etc.)

Tuesday:
Running/jogging for 30 minutes

Wednesday:
Go for a walk in a part of town with a lot of staircases, hill climbing, or a shopping mall with a lot of levels and take the stairs, walk for at least 30 minutes

Thursday:
Weight training or bodyweight exercises for at least 30 minutes

Friday:
Go for a walk around a new part of the city for at least 30 minutes

Saturday:
Bike riding around town for at least 30 minutes

Sunday:
Free choice day but for at least 30 minutes

Again, start slow, gradually increase, and have fun doing it! When it comes to weight training you don't need to be lifting a hundred pounds, just start with a weight amount that is easy to repeat but still gives you some resistance. Try for a weight that you can lift 10-12 times in a row before taking a break. This will allow you to work on your endurance while still building some muscle.

As with everything, take your time and try to focus on enjoying the various activities as much as possible to take the most benefit from the time spent.

Chapter 5:

Beginner Recipes to Soothe the Gut

You know the right foods to eat, but how can we incorporate them into everyday meals? Here are just a few ways to use the right foods to heal your gut.

Quinoa Chicken Dish

Ingredients

1 cup quinoa, washed or pre-washed
2 cup bone broth (or 1 ¾ cup hot water with 2 concentrate cubes of bone broth)
1 ½ cup of organic frozen vegetables
1 cup of cooked shredded or cubed organic chicken
1 tsp. garlic powder
1 tsp. onion powder
1 tsp. paprika
1 tsp. basil
1 tsp. salt
1 tsp. pepper
Sprouted beans or grains

Directions

Step 1: Boil the vegetables in a small pot until they are tender.

Step 2: Mix in the cooked chicken and set aside.

Step 3: Meanwhile combine the quinoa, bone broth, and seasonings in a separate pot. Stir until blended and bring to a boil.

Step 4: Reduce heat to low, cover and simmer for about 15 minutes or until the water had evaporated.

Step 5: Mix in the vegetable and chicken mixture and re-cover for another 5 minutes.

Step 6: Top with some sprouted beans or grains and enjoy!

Rice and Kimchi

Ingredients

1 cup brown rice
2 cups bone broth (or 1 ¾ cup hot water with 2 concentrate cubes of bone broth)
Organic Kimchi
Soy Sauce

Directions

Step 1: Boil the rice with the bone broth instead of water.

Step 2: When the rice is done, spoon some into a bowl.

Step 3: Mix in some kimchi.

Step 4: Season with some soy sauce.

Step 5: Serve.

This is a great light lunch / filling snack.

Mixed Sprouted Salad

Directions

Step 1: To begin with, use any sprouted lentils, nuts, seeds you want or have handy.

Step 2: Add any chopped vegetables you like such as tomatoes, avocados, carrots, peas, beans, green onions, red onions, cabbage, kohlrabi, pickled beets, etc.

Step 3: Homemade vinaigrette or ranch salad dressing.

Step 4: Toss together and enjoy as a light meal or as a quick side dish.

How to sprout your own lentils!

Ingredients

Lentils of choice
Water and a bowl big enough

Directions

Step 1: Put the lentils in a bowl and fill it with water until they are covered with 1-2 inches of water.

Step 2: Let them soak overnight.

Step 3: The next morning pour the bowl into a colander, rinse them and set on a plate.

Step 4: Cover them with a cloth and set aside.

Step 5: The next morning repeat the washing process and continue every morning until they are at your desired length.

Step 6: Store in the refrigerator for up to a few days and use to top all your favorite recipes, as a meat substitute in dishes, or eat straight as an awesome side dish.

Garlic Butter Sprouts

Ingredients

2 Tbsp. butter
2 Tbsp. coconut oil
1 finely chopped onion
5-8 cloves of minced garlic
1 small minced chili pepper (jalapeño, serrano, habanero)
¼ tsp. cayenne pepper
2 cups sprouted beans of your choice
3 Tbsp. bone broth
Toasted sesame oil

Directions

Step 1: In a pan, heat up 1 Tbsp. of butter and coconut oil on high for 1-2 minutes.

Step 2: Add garlic, onion, chili pepper, and cayenne and sauté for a minute (don't let it burn).

Step 3: Add the sprouts and stir for a minute.

Step 4: Add the bone broth, reduce the heat to low and simmer for 2-3 minutes.

Step 5: Take it off the burner and add 1 Tbsp. butter and stir well.

Step 6: Serve in dishes with rice, noodles, or quinoa and drizzle with sesame oil.

Coconut Curry

Ingredients

1 Tbsp. coconut oil
1 Tbsp. curry powder
½ cup onion, diced
1 Tbsp. grated ginger
4 minced cloves garlic
1 cup chicken bone broth
½ cup broccoli, diced
¼ cup tomato, diced
½ cup carrots, diced
⅓ cup snow peas
2 cans light coconut milk
Pinch cayenne pepper
Pinch sea salt and black pepper
1 cup quinoa, washed or pre-washed
1 (14-ounce) can of coconut milk
½ cup water or bone broth

Directions

Step 1: In a small pot toast the dry quinoa over medium heat for 2-3 minutes.

Step 2: Add one can of coconut milk and ½ cup of water or bone broth.

Step 3: Bring to a boil, reduce heat, cover and simmer for 15 minutes or until all the water is evaporated. Fluff with a fork and set aside.

Step 4: Meanwhile, heat a large pan over medium heat and toss in 1 Tbsp. of coconut oil.

Step 5: Add the ginger, carrot, garlic, broccoli, onions, and a pinch of salt and pepper. Stirring often, cook until the vegetables are softened, about 5 minutes.

Step 6: Add the curry powder, bone broth, cayenne pepper, coconut milk, and one more pinch of salt. Stir and bring to a simmer, reduce heat a little and cook for 10-15 minutes. While it is cooking, taste it for the flavor. If it's too sweet, add some cumin and turmeric, if it needs more spice, add another pinch of cayenne pepper, if it needs more warmth, add a pinch of cinnamon.

Step 7: Add the tomatoes and the snow peas in the last 5 minutes so they don't get mushy.

Step 8: Serve over coconut quinoa and top with lemon or lime juice and any herbs you want.

Chapter 6:
The Comprehensive Cure

Now let's put all the information discussed together and you'll have a powerful punch to healing your leaky gut syndrome! While lowering your stress, or eating better, or taking a few supplements will help, doing all of them will really tackle the illness and allow your body to get back on the right track as soon as possible and with no more questionable medications.

The Four Step Lifestyle Change

Step One:

Start by eliminating any cause that may have started the damage to your gut. If you suspect it was a medication, talk to your doctor about taking a different route with the regimen. Perhaps there is an alternative medicine that could be used or a different medicine that won't cause any damage to the stomach and intestines. If your doctor won't take your concerns about your stomach and well-being seriously, try getting a second opinion from a holistic doctor.

If you think the damage was caused by a certain toxin that was present in a favorite food of yours, try to find another version of that food, one that is more basic, less preserved, or grown locally. If you aren't sure exactly what started the damage, start by looking into any medications you are consistently taking, any consistently consumed food items, and anything that you eat from. If you still don't find anything out of the ordinary, start eating more wholesome foods that are free from flavorings, coloring, chemicals, preservatives, GMOs, hormones and antibiotics, and foods that have been processed.

Step Two:

Incorporate the healing foods listed in chapters 2 and 3 into your daily meals. Chapter 5 gives some tasty starter recipes, but you can replace ingredients in your favorite recipes with the super foods listed.

Whenever you eat a salad or casserole, toss some bean sprouts on top. Whenever you make a rice or quinoa dish, instead of using just plain water use a bone broth. It will add glorious flavor and a slew of gut-healing nutrients. Instead of using canola, vegetable, or olive oil, substitute them for coconut oil. It adds a wonderful flavor to dishes. Garlic can be added to virtually any meat or vegetable dish as well as many homemade breads and pasta dishes. Ginger can be added to many dishes as well and pairs extremely well with most Asian and pastry dishes. Kefir and yogurts make excellent breakfasts especially when paired with fruit or a hardboiled egg.

Also, fermented beverages like Kombucha are a good way to quit soda pop. They have the carbonation that can easily substitute soda and instead of drinking something that gives you no nutritional value whatsoever, you will be drinking something that will heal your body and provide you with nutrients that are sorely missing from our modern diets. Soon adding and substituting beneficial ingredients will be like second nature and you won't know how you ever enjoyed a meal before them!

Step Three:

Add supplements to your daily regimen. As stated throughout this book, our modern diets lack the nutrients, minerals, and vitamins that we need to thrive. While the type of basic food hasn't changed (beef, chicken, vegetables, fruits, fish, nuts, and so on) the way they are grown and raised has. Our food isn't as healthy and natural anymore and therefore we miss out on the many nutrients we need. Whether you start with a multivitamin or go with specific types of digestive enzymes or L-glutamine, adding supplements to your day will ensure you are getting the nutrients you need to heal and be healthy.

Step Four:

Finally, lowering your stress is beneficial all around. This one may be harder to do, as stressors are usually out of our control. However, how we react to them is somewhat within our control. While exercise uses up the hormones that were already released into your body after encountering a stressor, here are some things you can do in the moment when you are confronted with stress.

Meditate: Before you get amped up over a stressor, take a few minutes and find a quiet place. Sit down and focus on the present. Try to keep your mind neutral, don't think about the past or what might happen next, just breath in and breathe out. If you find your emotions leaking in, that's okay. However, instead of dwelling on the emotions, acknowledged them and move on. If you find your mind wandering to thoughts about the past or future, gently remind yourself to one back to the present and consciously follow your breathing; in and out, in and out.

Focus on your body: sit down in a chair and plant your feet flat on the ground. Imagine tiny holes in the soles of your feet. As you inhale imagine warm air flowing into the holes in your feet up through your ankles, then your calves, your knees and thighs, your pelvis and abdomen and up to your chest. When you exhale imagine the warm air leaving through the holes after traveling back down through your body.

You can also sit straight-backed, and start by focusing on the muscles in your neck. Tense them and then relax them. Move to your shoulders and upper back, tense the muscles there and then relax them. Next focus on your upper arms, lower arms, hands, abdomen and lower back, buttocks, upper legs and lower legs, and finally the feet. By consciously focusing on each muscle group, tensing them up and relaxing them, you may find that you have been tensing a certain muscle group the whole time, and the physical effort to tense and relax them will allow you to let go and return your body to its natural state.

Laugh it up: having a good chuckle is amazing for your mental health. It lowers cortisol (a hormone that is released when your body activates its stress response system) and releases endorphins (the feel-good chemical that makes you happy and manages pain). Take a few minutes to watch a funny video, read some comics, or talk to someone that makes your laugh.

Crank up the tunes: studies show that listening to soothing sounds can lower blood pressure, anxiety, and heart rate. Create a playlist with soft nature sounds and focus on the instruments or animals and water you hear.

By enacting these four steps into your everyday life will heal your gut and make you a healthier and happier person. You will be amazed how simple the changes will be and what a huge difference they make. Remember to always be conscious of where your food comes from and to have as much fun as possible. The greatest cure is happiness. Enjoy life and all it has to offer, love the people around you, forgive when you can, and lead a fun and active life!

Conclusion

Thanks for making it through to the end of this book, let's hope it was informative and able to provide you with all of the tools you need to achieve your goals whatever they may be.

Leaky gut syndrome is a common illness that can be disruptive, debilitating, and can lead to more serious conditions. This condition is something that is both very common and often overlooked. It has common symptoms but it has basic causes.

Now that you know what types of behaviors and foods can cause leaky gut, you have the advantage of recognizing the symptoms early on and fixing the issue before it gets out of hand.

If this is a condition that is already present, you now know what you can do about it and that you don't need to pay for expensive medicine to start the healing process, and you can start right now!

The next step is to start ridding your pantry and your meals of bad food. Anything that is heavily-processed, filled with preservatives, chemicals, flavorings and coloring, and many foods that come in boxes, bags, and cans. You know now where to source your meats as well and can make a more educated decision about what you put into your body.

You can also start exercising immediately by setting aside 30-60 minutes a day. Make a personal commitment to being active from today. It will help both mentally and physically to try and exercise at the same time every day. Mentally, you will be prepared to exercise and won't be spending time working up to the actual work out. Physically, your body will come to expect the exercise around the same time and the work will be less stressful.

Remember, start slow and gradually increase the amount whenever you start a new exercise. Going too fast or too far too soon will usually guarantee an injury, which will cause more stress on your body and mind. Plus, it may set you back on your road to recovery. Therefore, start slow and above all things, enjoy your workout! If you don't enjoy what you do, you won't continue it.

If one type of exercise doesn't work for you or it just completely bores you, find another type. Use YouTube as your free online resource to find alternative exciting exercises. There are so many things to do to be active and many ways to do them.

Remember the four-step lifestyle change: eliminate the cause if you know what it might be, readjust your diet to exclude harmful foods and incorporate beneficial foods, add some supplements that agree with your system and work for your needs, and try to decrease your stress levels with both exercise and calming techniques. This is the best and most natural way to heal your body, and it will thank you later on.

Maintain a healthy gut and a healthy immune system by keeping up these practices. You will notice other benefits as well such as weight loss, clearer skin, fewer headaches and migraines, better sleep, and more confidence. Something we could all use these days!

Finally, if you found this book useful in any way, a review online is always appreciated!

Don't forget to grab your FREE eBook before you leave

Visit the link below to get your free eBook now...
www.bit.ly/myvouchgift

101 Inspirational Cooking Quotes

Inside this free eBook, you will find fascinating cooking quotes from awe-inspiring people who love to cook just like you!

Ps. Feel free to share this free gift with your friends & family!